YOGA AT HOME

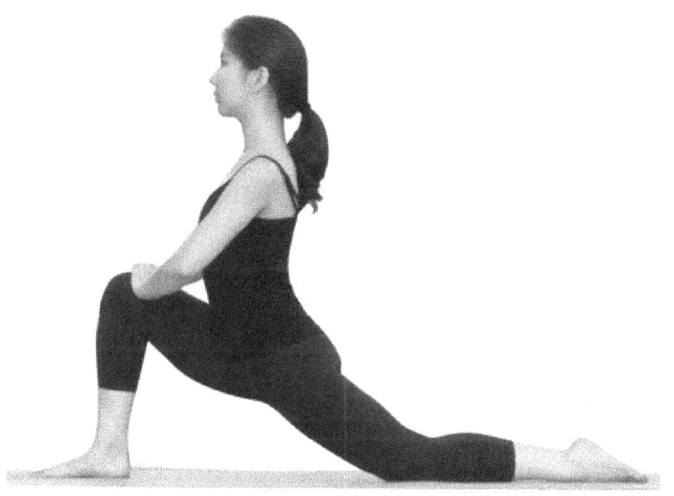

A Comprehensive Guide to 60 Plus Poses for Beginners and Intermediates, Including Benefits, Tips, and Health Enhancement Techniques

Tom M. Yukteswar

Table of Content

Chapter 1: Introduction

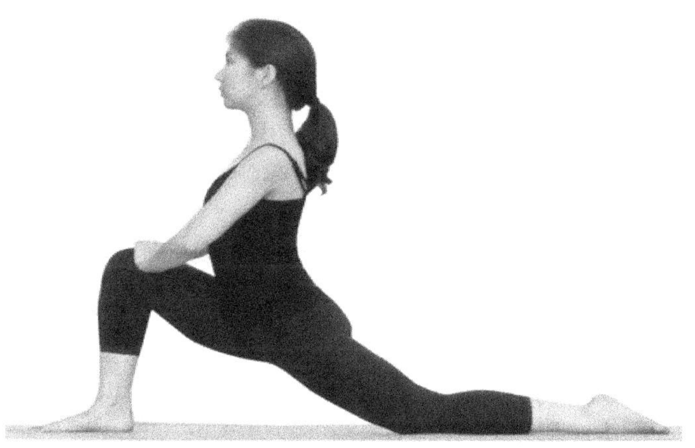

Welcome to''Yoga at Home: A Comprehensive
Guide to 60 Plus Poses for Beginners and
Intermediates, Including Benefits, Tips, and Health
Enhancement Techniques'' in this book, we embark
on a journey to explore the profound practice of
yoga, offering you a comprehensive guide to
enhance your physical and mental well-being from
the comfort of your own home.

The word *"yoga"* itself derives from *Sanskrit*, meaning "to join, unite, or yoke together," symbolizing the harmonious integration of various aspects of the self. Whether you're a beginner or an experienced yogi, the benefits of yoga are accessible to all, offering a path towards greater physical resilience and emotional balance.

Yoga is a holistic practice that integrates the mind, body, and spirit. Yoga's roots can be traced back thousands of years to ancient Eastern civilizations, originating in ancient India, its popularity has surged in the modern Western world. What was once perceived as an esoteric practice reserved for ascetics and spiritual seekers has evolved into a mainstream lifestyle choice for individuals seeking balance and well-being. Yoga has transcended cultural boundaries to become a globally recognized method for achieving inner harmony and physical vitality.

From serene outdoor retreats to bustling urban studios, yoga has found its place in diverse settings, catering to practitioners of all backgrounds and experiences. Whether practicing amidst nature's tranquility or within the confines of a contemporary studio, the essence of yoga remains constant – a journey towards self-discovery and inner peace.

Yoga encompasses guidance on healthy living, nutrition, and cultivating a positive mindset. It is an approach to wellness that extends beyond the mat and into everyday life. Central to the philosophy of yoga is the belief in the interconnectedness of all aspects of existence – the mind, body, and spirit. Through the practice of yoga, individuals seek to bridge these elements, fostering a sense of unity and wholeness within themselves.

As we delve into the depths of yoga in this book, remember that yoga is not about perfection but about exploration and self-discovery. Whether you're stepping onto the mat for the first time or deepening your practice, embrace the journey with an open heart and mind.

Chapter 2:
Yoga for All

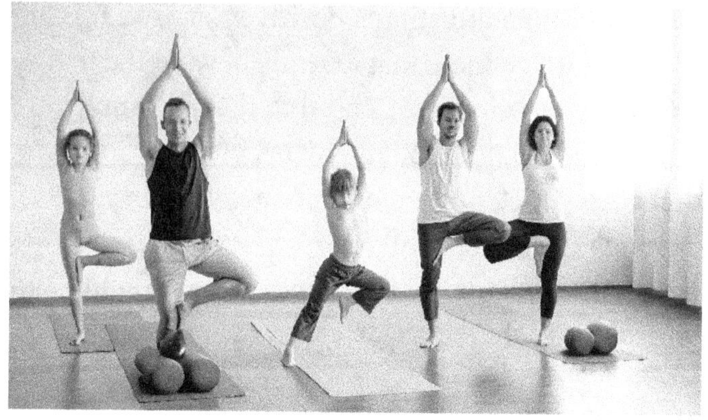

Yoga is a practice for everyone, regardless of age, fitness level, or physical condition. Whether you're young or old, injured or fit, flexible or inflexible, male or female, there is always a suitable way for you to engage in yoga. In this book, we explore the inclusive nature of yoga and the accessibility of its practice to Beginners and Intermediates.

One of the remarkable aspects of yoga is its universality. While some advanced poses may appear daunting, the vast majority of yoga postures are accessible to beginners. With an appropriate guideline, most people can begin their yoga journey regardless of their starting point.

Finding Your Path

In the world of yoga, there is a myriad of styles and approaches, ensuring that there is something for everyone. Whether you're drawn to the gentle flow of Hatha yoga, the dynamic sequences of Vinyasa, or the precise alignment of Iyengar yoga, there is a practice suited to your preferences and needs.

Chapter 3: Types of Yoga

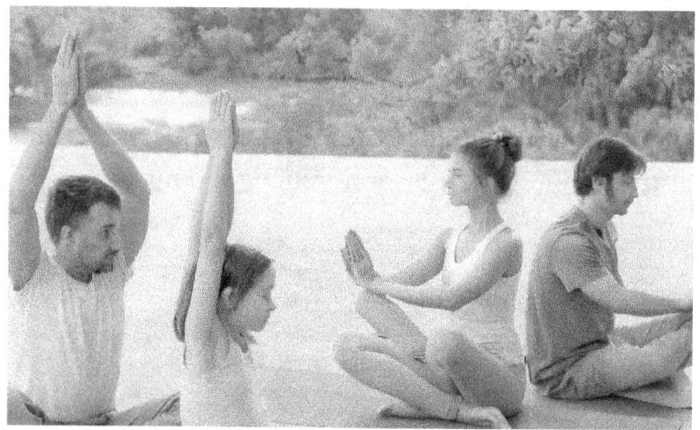

1. Hatha Yoga:

Hatha yoga is a foundational style that focuses on physical postures (asanas) and breathing techniques (pranayama). It is often considered a gentle form of yoga and is suitable for beginners.

- Benefits: Increases flexibility, improves balance, enhances relaxation, promotes stress relief, and builds strength.

- Suitable for: Beginners and all levels.
- Level: Beginner to intermediate.

2. Vinyasa Yoga:

Vinyasa yoga emphasizes the coordination of movement with breath, creating a fluid and dynamic practice. It involves flowing sequences of poses linked together in a continuous and rhythmic manner.

- Benefits: Builds cardiovascular health, increases flexibility, improves strength and endurance, enhances mental focus, and promotes stress reduction.

- Suitable for: Those seeking a dynamic and challenging practice.
- Level: Beginner to advanced.

3. Ashtanga Yoga:

Ashtanga yoga is a rigorous and structured practice that follows a specific sequence of poses. It involves synchronized breathing and progressive series of postures designed to build strength, flexibility, and stamina.

- Benefits: Builds strength, improves flexibility, enhances stamina and endurance, promotes detoxification, and increases mental focus and discipline.

- Suitable for: Those seeking a structured and rigorous practice.
- Level: Intermediate to advanced.

4. Iyengar Yoga:

Iyengar yoga places emphasis on precision and alignment in each pose. Props such as blocks, straps, and bolsters are often used to assist practitioners in achieving proper alignment and depth in their poses.

- Benefits: Improves alignment and posture, increases flexibility, enhances strength and stability, promotes injury recovery, and cultivates body awareness.

- Suitable for: Individuals with specific alignment needs or those recovering from injuries.
- Level: Beginner to advanced.

5. Bikram Yoga:

Bikram yoga, also known as hot yoga, is practiced in a heated room with temperatures typically ranging from 95 to 105 degrees Fahrenheit. It follows a set sequence of 26 poses and two breathing exercises, intended to promote detoxification and flexibility.

- Benefits: Increases flexibility, promotes detoxification through sweating, enhances cardiovascular health, improves stamina, and aids weight loss.

- Suitable for: Those comfortable with heat and seeking a challenging physical practice.
- Level: Beginner to intermediate.

6. Kundalini Yoga:

Kundalini yoga incorporates dynamic movements, breathing techniques, chanting, and meditation to awaken the energy at the base of the spine (kundalini). It aims to release energy blockages and promote spiritual growth.

- Benefits: Activates energy centers, promotes spiritual growth and self-awareness, enhances emotional balance, reduces stress and anxiety, and improves overall vitality.

- Suitable for: Those seeking a spiritual and transformative practice.
- Level: Beginner to advanced.

7. Yin Yoga:

Yin yoga focuses on passive, long-held poses that target the deep connective tissues of the body. It encourages relaxation and flexibility, often incorporating mindfulness and meditation practices.

- Benefits: Increases flexibility and joint mobility, releases tension in deep connective tissues, promotes relaxation and stress reduction, improves circulation, and enhances mindfulness.

- Suitable for: Individuals looking to balance out a more active yoga practice or those with tight muscles and joints.
- Level: Beginner to advanced.

8. Restorative Yoga:

Restorative yoga involves gentle poses supported by props, allowing the body to deeply relax and restore. It is particularly beneficial for reducing stress, promoting healing, and cultivating a sense of well-being.

- Benefits: Promotes deep relaxation and stress relief, aids in injury recovery, enhances flexibility and joint mobility, improves sleep quality, and cultivates a sense of well-being.

- Suitable for: Individuals recovering from injuries, those experiencing high levels of stress, or anyone seeking gentle relaxation.
- Level: Beginner to advanced.

9. Power Yoga:

Power yoga is a dynamic and athletic style influenced by Ashtanga yoga. It emphasizes strength, endurance, and flexibility through a fast-paced practice that may vary in sequence and intensity.

- Benefits: Builds strength, increases cardiovascular fitness, improves flexibility and endurance, enhances mental focus and concentration, and promotes weight loss.

- Suitable for: Those seeking a challenging and dynamic practice.
- Level: Intermediate to advanced.

10. Yoga Nidra:

Yoga Nidra, also known as yogic sleep, is a guided meditation technique that induces deep relaxation and inner awareness. Practitioners are led through a systematic process of relaxation, visualization, and self-inquiry to achieve a state of profound relaxation and heightened consciousness.

- Benefits: Induces deep relaxation and stress reduction, promotes better sleep quality, enhances self-awareness and inner peace, reduces anxiety and depression, and supports emotional healing.

- Suitable for: Anyone seeking deep relaxation and a meditative experience.
- Level: Beginner to advanced.

Each yoga styles listed above provide unique benefits and approaches to physical, mental, and spiritual well-being. Exploring different styles can help individuals find the practice that best suits their needs and preferences.

The benefits and recommendations listed serve as general guidelines, and individuals should listen to their bodies and consult with a qualified yoga instructor to determine the most appropriate practice for their needs and abilities.

Chapter 4:
Health Benefit of Yoga

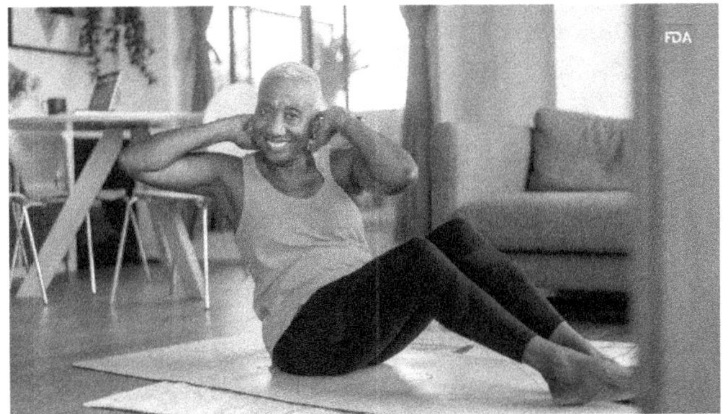

1. Improved posture:

Yoga encourages proper alignment and strengthens the muscles that support the spine, resulting in improved posture. By practicing yoga poses that emphasize lengthening the spine and opening the chest, individuals can correct postural imbalances and alleviate discomfort associated with poor posture.

2. Better sleep:

Regular practice of yoga has been shown to improve sleep quality by promoting relaxation, reducing stress and anxiety levels, and calming the nervous system. By incorporating gentle yoga stretches and relaxation techniques before bedtime, individuals can create a conducive environment for restful sleep.

3. Increased natural energy level and vitality:

Yoga helps to release tension and increase circulation throughout the body, resulting in a boost in natural energy levels and vitality. By practicing invigorating yoga sequences and breathwork techniques, individuals can awaken their energy centers and cultivate a sense of vibrancy and vitality.

4. Greater flexibility, strength, and stamina:

Yoga poses target all major muscle groups, promoting greater flexibility, strength, and stamina. Through regular practice, individuals can gradually increase their range of motion, build muscle strength, and enhance their endurance, leading to improved physical performance and resilience.

5. Better balance:

Yoga poses that focus on stability and proprioception help to improve balance and coordination. By practicing standing balances and poses that challenge equilibrium, individuals can enhance their proprioceptive awareness and reduce the risk of falls and injuries.

6. Stronger immune system:

Yoga practice stimulates the lymphatic system and promotes detoxification, leading to a stronger immune response. By incorporating yoga poses that involve gentle twists and inversions, individuals can support lymphatic drainage and enhance immune function.

7. Pulse and respiratory rate decreases:

Through deep breathing exercises and relaxation techniques, yoga practice can lower both pulse and respiratory rates. By focusing on slow, rhythmic breathing, individuals can activate the parasympathetic nervous system, promoting relaxation and reducing stress levels.

8. Blood pressure decreases:

Yoga practice has been shown to reduce blood pressure levels by promoting relaxation, improving circulation, and reducing stress. By incorporating yoga poses that emphasize gentle stretching and deep breathing, individuals can support cardiovascular health and lower blood pressure.

9. Cardiovascular efficiency increases:

Dynamic yoga sequences and aerobic practices like Vinyasa yoga can improve cardiovascular efficiency by increasing heart rate and circulation. By engaging in regular cardiovascular-focused yoga practices, individuals can enhance heart health and improve overall cardiovascular function.

10. Respiratory efficiency increases:

Breath-focused yoga practices, such as pranayama, improve respiratory efficiency by increasing lung capacity and strengthening respiratory muscles. By practicing breath control techniques and mindful breathing, individuals can optimize oxygen intake and enhance respiratory function.

11. Cholesterol decreases:

Yoga practice, combined with a healthy lifestyle, can help lower cholesterol levels by promoting weight management, reducing stress, and improving circulation. By incorporating yoga poses that support cardiovascular health and metabolic function, individuals can maintain healthy cholesterol levels.

12. Cleansing and regulating of all the body's systems:

Yoga practice stimulates the body's natural detoxification processes and supports the optimal functioning of all bodily systems. By practicing yoga poses that stimulate digestion, circulation, and lymphatic drainage, individuals can promote overall health and well-being.

13. Calm and clarity:

Yoga promotes a sense of inner calm and mental clarity through mindfulness and relaxation techniques.

14. Increased awareness of body and movement:

Yoga enhances body awareness and promotes mindful movement, helping individuals develop a deeper connection with their physical selves.

15. Promoting better breathing:

Yoga emphasizes conscious breathing techniques that promote deep, diaphragmatic breathing and enhance respiratory function. By practicing breath work exercises and focusing on breath awareness, individuals can improve lung capacity and optimize oxygen intake.

Chapter 5:
Risk and Side Effects

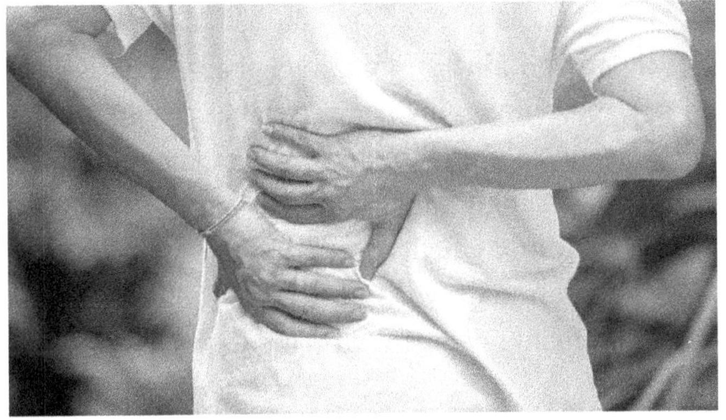

In our exploration of yoga's transformative power, it's essential to acknowledge that, like any physical activity, there are potential risks and side effects associated with yoga practice. While yoga is generally safe for most people, it's essential to be informed about these risks to practice safely and responsibly. In this chapter, we delve into common risks and side effects of yoga, along with strategies to minimize them.

1. **Musculoskeletal Injuries:** Performing yoga poses incorrectly or pushing beyond your limits can lead to musculoskeletal injuries

such as strains, sprains, or overuse injuries. It's crucial to practice proper alignment and listen to your body's signals to prevent injury.

2. **Joint Pain:** Certain yoga poses, especially those involving deep stretches or extreme ranges of motion, may exacerbate joint pain, particularly in individuals with pre-existing conditions such as arthritis or joint hypermobility. Modifications and props can help alleviate strain on the joints.

3. **Overexertion**: Pushing too hard or practicing intense yoga styles without adequate rest can lead to overexertion, fatigue, and burnout. It's essential to balance challenging practices with restorative and gentle sessions to prevent exhaustion.

4. **Heat-Related Issues:** Practicing hot yoga in a heated room can increase the risk of dehydration, heat exhaustion, or heat stroke, especially in individuals with certain medical conditions or those unaccustomed to high temperatures. Staying hydrated and

taking breaks as needed is crucial in hot yoga classes.

5. **Preexisting Conditions:** Individuals with preexisting medical conditions, such as musculoskeletal disorders, cardiovascular issues, or neurological conditions, may be more susceptible to injury or adverse reactions during yoga practice. It is important for such individuals to consult with a healthcare professional before beginning a yoga program and to practice under the guidance of a qualified instructor.

6. **Psychological Distress:** Yoga practice, particularly when combined with breath work and meditation, can sometimes trigger emotional or psychological distress in individuals with underlying trauma or mental health issues. It is essential for practitioners to approach yoga practice with self-awareness and to seek support if needed.

Chapter 6:
Managing Side Effects

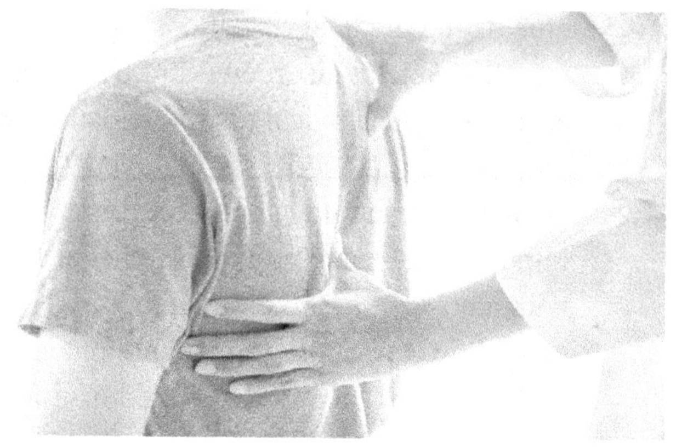

1. **Listen to Your Body:** Pay attention to your body's signals during yoga practice. If a pose feels uncomfortable or painful, back off or modify it to suit your needs. Pushing through pain can lead to injury.

2. **Modify as Needed:** Don't hesitate to modify poses or use props such as blocks, straps, or blankets to support your practice. Modifying poses allows you to adapt to your body's limitations and prevent strain or injury.

3. **Stay Hydrated:** Drink plenty of water before, during, and after yoga practice, especially in hot or intense classes. Proper hydration is essential for maintaining energy levels and preventing heat-related issues.

4. **Take Rest Days:** Incorporate rest days into your yoga routine to allow your body time to recover and prevent overuse injuries. Restorative practices such as gentle stretching or meditation can promote relaxation and recovery.

5. **Practice Mindful Breathing:** Incorporate mindful breathing techniques to regulate your body's response to stress and exertion. Deep, diaphragmatic breathing can help reduce tension and promote relaxation during practice.

6. **Choose the Right Style:** Select a yoga style and class level that aligns with your current fitness level, goals, and preferences. Avoid advanced classes or challenging poses if you are new to yoga or have limited experience.

7. By practicing yoga mindfully, listening to your body, and seeking guidance from qualified instructors, you can minimize the risks associated with yoga practice and enjoy its numerous benefits safely and effectively. Remember that yoga is a journey of self-discovery and self-care, and prioritizing your well-being is paramount.

Chapter 7:
Steps to Start a Home Yoga Practice

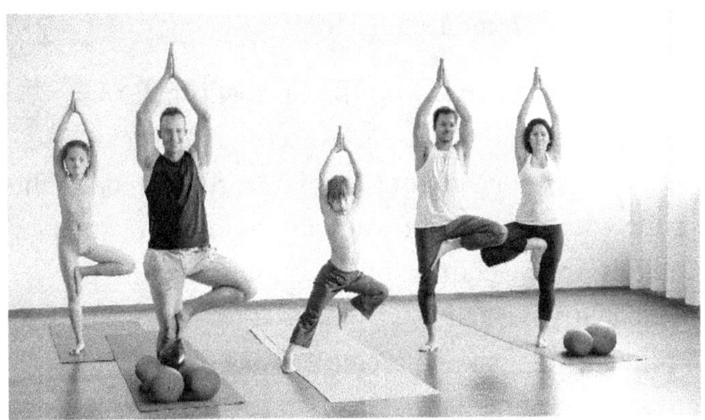

Embarking on a home yoga practice can be a rewarding journey towards physical, mental, and spiritual well-being. In this chapter, we provide a comprehensive guide to help you establish and sustain a fulfilling yoga practice within the comfort of your own home.

1. Set Your Intention

Before beginning your home yoga practice, take a moment to reflect on your intentions and goals. Consider what you hope to achieve through yoga, whether it's increasing flexibility, reducing stress, or cultivating mindfulness. Setting a clear intention will guide your practice and help you stay focused and motivated.

2. Create a Dedicated Space

Designate a space in your home specifically for yoga practice. Ideally, choose a quiet, clutter-free area with enough room to move freely. Decorate the space with items that inspire and uplift you, such as candles, incense, or inspiring quotes. Having a dedicated yoga space will make it easier to establish a regular practice and create a sense of sacredness around your practice.

3. Gather Your Equipment

You don't need fancy equipment to practice yoga at home, but having a few essential items can enhance your practice. Invest in a quality yoga mat that provides cushioning and support for your joints. You may also want to have props such as blocks, straps, and bolsters on hand to assist with alignment and deepen your practice.

4. Choose Your Practice Time

Select a time of day that works best for you to establish a consistent yoga routine. Whether it's first thing in the morning to set a positive tone for the day, during your lunch break to re-energize and de-stress, or in the evening to unwind and relax, find a time that aligns with your schedule and preferences. Consistency is key to building a sustainable home yoga practice.

5. Start with Simple Sequences

Begin your home yoga practice with simple sequences that focus on foundational poses and basic movements. Start with gentle warm-up poses to awaken your body and connect with your breath, then gradually progress to more challenging poses as your practice evolves. Listen to your body and honor its limitations, modifying poses as needed to suit your individual needs and abilities.

6. Cultivate Self-Discipline and Compassion

Consistency and self-discipline are essential for maintaining a home yoga practice. Set realistic goals for yourself and commit to practicing regularly, even on days when you don't feel motivated. Be gentle and compassionate with yourself, understanding that progress takes time and that it's okay to take breaks or modify your practice as needed.

7. Listen to Your Body

Above all, listen to your body and trust your intuition. Pay attention to how different poses and sequences make you feel physically, mentally, and emotionally. If something doesn't feel right, don't push through it. Take a step back, modify the pose, or skip it altogether. Your body knows best, so honor its wisdom and practice with mindfulness and self-awareness.

By following these steps and embracing the journey with an open heart and mind, you can establish a fulfilling home yoga practice that nourishes your body, mind, and spirit. Remember that yoga is a personal and transformative journey, and the most important thing is to show up on your mat with sincerity and intention, ready to embrace the present moment with awareness and compassion.

Chapter 8:
Materials Needed for Practice

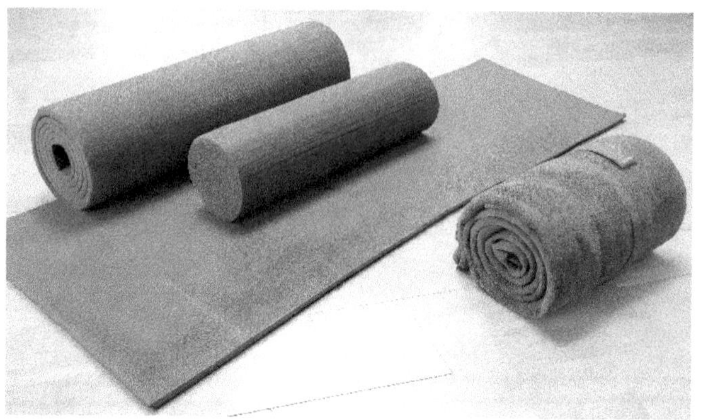

In this chapter, we explore the essential materials and equipment that will enhance your yoga practice and create a supportive environment for your journey of self-discovery and self-care. From yoga mats to props and accessories, having the right tools at your disposal can significantly enhance your comfort, safety, and enjoyment during yoga practice.

1. Yoga Mat

A yoga mat is perhaps the most essential piece of equipment for any yoga practitioner. It provides a stable and comfortable surface for practicing yoga poses, protecting your joints and preventing slipping. When choosing a yoga mat, look for one that offers adequate cushioning, traction, and durability to support your practice. Consider factors such as thickness, material, and texture to find a mat that suits your needs and preferences.

2. Yoga Props

Yoga props are versatile tools that can support proper alignment, enhance stability, and deepen your practice. Some essential yoga props include:

- **Yoga Blocks:** Blocks are rectangular foam or cork blocks that provide support and stability in standing, seated, and reclining poses. They can be used to modify poses, improve alignment, and increase accessibility for practitioners of all levels.

- **Yoga Straps:** Straps are adjustable bands that assist with stretching and deepening flexibility in yoga poses. They can be looped around the feet, hands, or body to extend reach and provide support in poses that require extra length or mobility.

- **Yoga Bolsters:** Bolsters are cylindrical or rectangular cushions that provide support and comfort in restorative and yin yoga poses. They can be used to elevate the hips, support the spine, and promote relaxation and release in passive poses.

- **Yoga Blankets:** Blankets are versatile props that can be used for additional support, cushioning, or warmth during yoga practice. They can be folded or rolled to provide padding under sensitive areas or to modify the height or angle of poses.

3. Yoga Towel

A yoga towel is a moisture-wicking towel designed to absorb sweat and provide traction on your yoga mat. It can help prevent slipping and sliding during intense or heated yoga practices, keeping you stable and focused throughout your practice. Look for a yoga towel that is lightweight, quick-drying, and machine washable for easy maintenance.

4. Yoga Mat Cleaner

Yoga mat cleaner is a natural cleaning solution specifically formulated to cleanse and disinfect your yoga mat. Regularly cleaning your yoga mat helps remove sweat, dirt, and bacteria, prolonging its lifespan and maintaining hygiene. Choose a mat cleaner that is non-toxic, eco-friendly, and free from harsh chemicals to ensure the safety of both you and your mat.

5. Comfortable Clothing

Comfortable clothing that allows for ease of movement is essential for a successful yoga practice. Choose breathable, moisture-wicking fabrics that stretch and move with your body, such as yoga leggings, shorts, or tank tops. Avoid restrictive or constricting clothing that may impede your range of motion or distract you during practice.

6. Water Bottle

Staying hydrated is crucial during yoga practice, especially in heated or intense classes. Keep a reusable water bottle nearby to sip on throughout your practice and stay hydrated and energized. Choose a durable, BPA-free water bottle that is easy to carry and refill, ensuring that you have access to fresh water whenever you need it.

7. Meditation Cushion (Optional)

If you incorporate meditation into your yoga practice, a meditation cushion or bolster can provide support and comfort during seated meditation sessions. Choose a cushion that is firm yet comfortable and offers proper alignment and elevation for your hips and spine. Alternatively, you can use a folded blanket or yoga block as a makeshift meditation cushion if needed.

By gathering these essential materials and equipment, you can create a supportive and inviting space for your home yoga practice, ensuring that you have everything you need to explore and deepen your yoga journey with comfort, safety, and ease.

Chapter 9:
Create Your Yoga Space
at Home

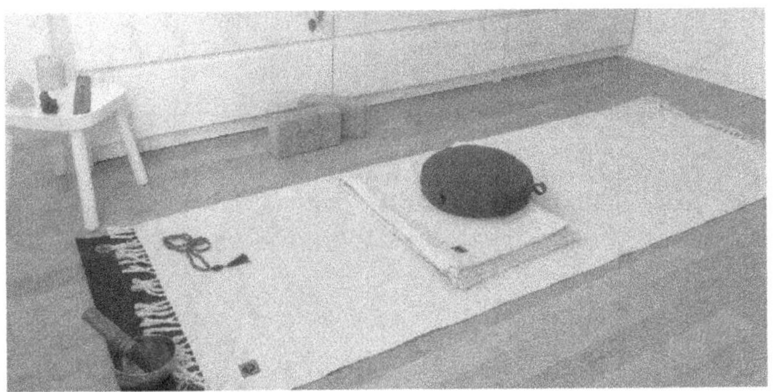

In this chapter, we delve into the process of designing and cultivating a dedicated yoga space within your home. By creating a tranquil and inspiring environment for your yoga practice, you can enhance your overall experience and foster a deeper connection with yourself and your practice.

1. Choose the Right Location

Selecting the ideal location for your home yoga space is the first step in creating a nurturing environment for your practice. Consider the following factors when choosing a space:

a. Quietness: Choose a quiet area of your home where you can practice without distractions or interruptions.

b. Natural Light: Opt for a space with ample natural light to create a bright and uplifting atmosphere for your practice. Position your yoga mat near a window or in a sunlit corner to benefit from natural daylight.

c. Ventilation: Ensure that the space is well-ventilated and free from stuffiness or odors. Good airflow will help keep you comfortable and refreshed during your practice.

d. Clutter-Free: Clear the space of clutter and unnecessary distractions to create a clean and serene environment. Remove any furniture or objects that may obstruct your movement or disrupt your focus.

2. Set the Ambiance

Once you've chosen your yoga space, it's time to set the ambiance and create a soothing atmosphere conducive to relaxation and introspection. Consider the following elements to enhance the ambiance of your yoga space:

a. Aromatherapy: Use essential oils or incense to infuse the space with calming and invigorating scents. Choose fragrances such as lavender, eucalyptus, or sandalwood to promote relaxation and focus during your practice.

b. Soft Lighting: Install soft lighting fixtures or use candles to create a warm and inviting atmosphere. Avoid harsh overhead lighting and opt for gentle, diffused light sources that promote a sense of tranquility.

c. Decorative Elements: Personalize your yoga space with decorative elements that inspire and uplift you. Incorporate items such as plants, artwork, or inspirational quotes to infuse the space with positive energy and intention.

d. Music or Soundscape: Play soft music or nature sounds to enhance the ambiance and deepen your immersion in the practice. Choose calming instrumental music or ambient sounds such as ocean waves or birdsong to create a serene auditory backdrop for your practice.

3. Organize Your Equipment

Keep your yoga equipment organized and readily accessible to streamline your practice and minimize distractions. Consider the following tips for organizing your yoga space:

a. Yoga Mat Storage: Invest in a yoga mat rack or storage bag to keep your yoga mat neatly rolled and out of the way when not in use.

b. Prop Storage: Store yoga props such as blocks, straps, and bolsters in a designated storage bin or shelf within arm's reach of your yoga mat.

c. Water Bottle Holder: Install a water bottle holder or keep a reusable water bottle

nearby to stay hydrated throughout your
practice.

d. Meditation Cushion: If you use a meditation
cushion or bolster, keep it within easy reach
for seated meditation sessions.

4. Create a Ritual

Establishing a ritual or routine before and after your
yoga practice can help you transition into and out of
the practice with mindfulness and intention.
Consider incorporating the following rituals into
your yoga space:

a. Mindfulness Practice: Begin each practice
with a few moments of mindfulness or
meditation to center yourself and set a
positive intention for your practice.

b. Breath work: Practice deep, conscious
breathing exercises such as pranayama to
calm the mind and connect with the present
moment.

c. Gratitude Practice: End each practice with a
    moment of gratitude, reflecting on the
    blessings and lessons of the day and
    expressing gratitude for the opportunity to
    practice yoga.

By creating a dedicated yoga space within your
home and infusing it with intention, mindfulness,
and positive energy, you can cultivate a sanctuary
for your practice and deepen your connection with
yoga as a transformative and healing practice. Take
the time to nurture and care for your yoga space,
and it will in turn nourish and support you on your
journey of self-discovery and self-care.

Chapter 10: Warming Up

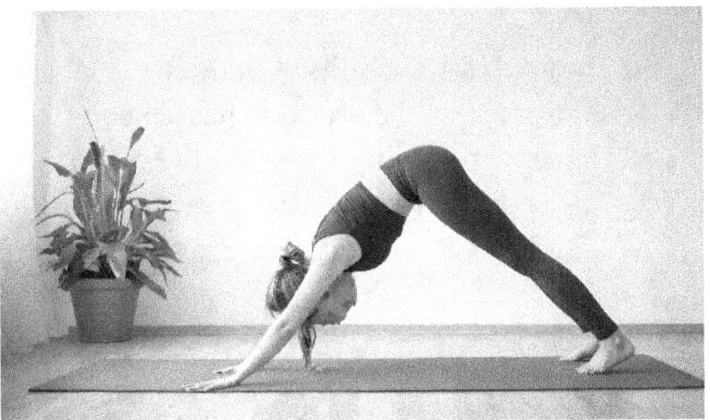

Warming up is an essential component of any yoga practice, preparing the body and mind for the physical and mental demands of asana (posture) practice. In this chapter, we explore the importance of warming up before yoga, along with a variety of effective warm-up sequences to help you start your practice with intention, mindfulness, and ease.

Importance of Warming Up

Warming up serves several important purposes in yoga practice:

Prevention of Injury: Warming up gradually increases blood flow to the muscles, joints, and connective tissues, reducing the risk of injury during more intense or challenging poses.

- **Improved Flexibility:** Gentle stretching and movement in the warm-up phase help increase flexibility and range of motion in the body, making it easier to move into deeper poses safely and effectively.

- **Mental Preparation:** Warming up allows you to transition from the busyness of daily life to a more focused and present state of mind, preparing you mentally for the practice ahead.

- **Enhanced Breath Awareness:** The warm-up phase provides an opportunity to synchronize movement with breath, cultivating awareness of the breath and promoting a sense of calm and centeredness.

Components of a Warm-Up Sequence

A well-rounded warm-up sequence typically includes the following components:

- **Gentle Movement:** Begin with gentle movements such as neck rolls, shoulder shrugs, and wrist circles to loosen up tight muscles and joints.

- **Dynamic Stretching:** Incorporate dynamic stretches that move the body through its full range of motion, such as forward folds, lunges, and twists, to increase flexibility and mobility.

- **Breath work:** Integrate breath work exercises such as ujjayi pranayama (victorious breath) or kapalabhati (skull shining breath) to deepen your breath awareness and activate the parasympathetic nervous system.

- **Sun Salutations (Surya Namaskar):** Sun salutations are a dynamic sequence of yoga poses that link movement with breath, providing a comprehensive warm-up for the entire body while building strength and stamina.

Chapter 11:
Warm-Up Sequences

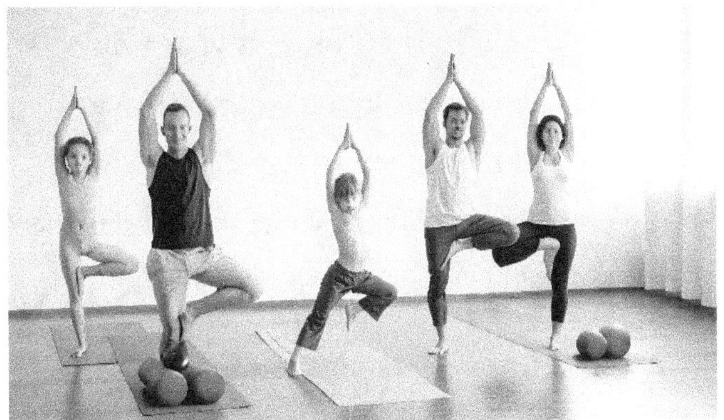

Warming up is a crucial aspect of yoga practice that prepares the body and mind for the deeper exploration of asana, breath work, and meditation. By incorporating gentle movement, dynamic stretching, breath awareness, and sun salutations into your warm-up routine, you can optimize the benefits of your yoga practice and cultivate a mindful and integrated approach to wellness. Remember to honor your body's needs and limitations, modifying poses as needed to ensure a safe and effective warm-up experience.

Sequence 1: Gentle Warm-Up

1. Seated Neck Rolls:

- Sit comfortably with a tall spine.
- Drop your right ear towards your right shoulder and gently roll your head in a circular motion, bringing your chin towards your chest and then over to the left shoulder.
- Repeat in the opposite direction.

2. Cat-Cow Stretch:

- Come to a tabletop position on hands and knees.
- Inhale, arch your back, and lift your chest and tailbone towards the ceiling (Cow Pose).
- Exhale, round your spine, and tuck your chin towards your chest (Cat Pose).
- Flow between Cat and Cow poses with each breath for several rounds.

3. **Downward Facing Dog:**

- From tabletop position, tuck your toes under, lift your hips towards the ceiling, and straighten your arms and legs, coming into an inverted V-shape.
- Pedal your feet and walk your hands out to stretch through the back of the legs and spine.

4. **Forward Fold:**

- From Downward Facing Dog, step your feet towards your hands at the top of your mat.
- Fold forward at the hips, allowing your head and torso to hang heavy.
- Bend your knees as much as needed to release tension in the hamstrings.

5. **Standing Side Stretch:**

- Come to standing, feet hip-width apart.

- ℘ Reach your arms overhead, interlace your fingers, and press your palms towards the ceiling.
- ℘ Lean gently to the right, stretching through the left side of the body.
- ℘ Hold for a few breaths, then switch sides.

Sequence 2: Hip Opening Flow

6. **Child's Pose (Balasana):**
- ℘ Start in a kneeling position, then sit back on your heels and fold forward, reaching your arms out in front of you.
- ℘ Rest your forehead on the mat and relax your hips towards your heels.

7. **Thread the Needle:**

- From tabletop, reach your right arm under your left arm, threading it through the space between your left hand and knee.
- Rest your right shoulder and ear on the mat.
- Hold for a few breaths, then switch sides.

8. Low Lunge (Anjaneyasana):

- Step your right foot forward between your hands and lower your left knee to the mat.
- Sink your hips down and forward, feeling a stretch in the front of your left hip.
- Repeat on the other side.

9. Happy Baby Pose (Ananda Balasana):

- Lie on your back and draw your knees towards your chest.
- Grab the outer edges of your feet with your hands and gently pull your knees towards the floor, opening your hips.

Sequence 3: Shoulder Mobility Flow

10. Shoulder Rolls:

- Stand tall with your arms by your sides.
- Inhale, shrug your shoulders up towards your ears, then exhale, roll them back and down.
- Repeat for several rounds, then switch directions.

11. Eagle Arms:

- Extend your arms out to the sides at shoulder height.
- Cross your right arm over your left, bringing your elbows together and wrapping your forearms around each other.
- Lift your elbows and press your palms together.

- ℘ Hold for a few breaths, then switch sides.

12. Neck Stretches:

- ℘ Drop your right ear towards your right shoulder and gently press down with your right hand, feeling a stretch along the left side of your neck.
- ℘ Hold for a few breaths, then switch sides.

13. Cow Face Arms:

- ℘ Reach your right arm up towards the ceiling, then bend your elbow and reach your right hand down your back.
- ℘ Reach your left arm behind you and bend your elbow, reaching your left hand up your back.
- ℘ Clasp your hands together if possible.
- ℘ Hold for a few breaths, then switch sides.

14. Supported Fish Pose (Matsyasana):

- ✍ Sit on the floor with your legs extended and place a yoga block or bolster behind you, horizontally along your mid-back.
- ✍ Lower your back onto the support and allow your arms to rest comfortably at your sides.
- ✍ Relax and breathe deeply, feeling a gentle opening in your chest and shoulders.

Sequence 4: Core Activation Flow

15. Boat Pose (Navasana):
- ✍ Sit on the mat with your knees bent and feet flat on the floor.
- ✍ Lean back slightly, engage your core, and lift your feet off the ground.
- ✍ Extend your arms forward parallel to the floor. Hold for a few breaths, then release.

16. Plank Pose:

- Come to a high plank position with your wrists directly under your shoulders and your body in a straight line from head to heels.
- Engage your core and hold for 30-60 seconds, breathing steadily.

17. Side Plank Pose (Vasisthasana):

- Shift your weight onto your right hand and outer edge of your right foot, stacking your left foot on top of your right.
- Extend your left arm towards the ceiling, creating a straight line from your head to your heels.
- Hold for a few breaths, then switch sides.

18. Supine Leg Lifts:

- Lie on your back with your arms by your sides.
- Lift your legs off the floor and extend them towards the ceiling. Lower them towards the

floor, keeping your lower back pressed into the mat.

- ℘ Lift them back up to the starting position.
- ℘ Repeat for several rounds.

Sequence 5: Spinal Mobility Flow

19. Seated Spinal Twists:

- ℘ Sit on the mat with your legs extended in front of you.
- ℘ Bend your right knee and cross it over your left leg, placing your right foot on the floor outside your left thigh.
- ℘ Inhale, lengthen your spine, and exhale, twist to the right, placing your left elbow on the outside of your right knee.
- ℘ Hold for a few breaths, then switch sides.

20. Sphinx Pose (Salamba Bhujangasana):

- ℘ Lie on your stomach with your elbows under your shoulders and forearms on the mat.
- ℘ Press into your forearms and lift your chest off the mat, lengthening through your spine.
- ℘ Hold for a few breaths, then release.

21. Dynamic Low Lunge:

- ℘ From Forward Fold, step your right foot back into a low lunge. Inhale, lift your arms overhead, and exhale, lower your hands to the mat.
- ℘ Repeat for several rounds, moving with your breath. Then switch sides.

Chapter 12

Yoga for Beginners

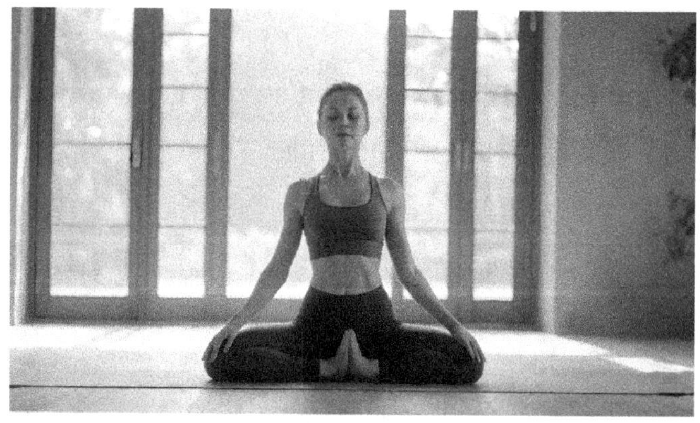

In this chapter, we will introduce beginners to the practice of yoga, providing guidance, tips, and foundational techniques to help you embark on your yoga journey with confidence and ease. Whether you're completely new to yoga or have dabbled in it before, this chapter will serve as a comprehensive starting point for developing a sustainable and fulfilling yoga practice.

1. Mountain Pose (Tadasana)

Guidelines:

- Stand tall with your feet hip-width apart, toes pointing forward.
- Engage your thigh muscles, lift your kneecaps, and gently tuck your tailbone.
- Roll your shoulders back and down, lengthen your spine, and reach your arms alongside your body with palms facing forward.

Benefits:

- Improves posture and alignment.
- Builds strength and stability in the legs, core, and back.
- Promotes focus and concentration.

Tips:

- Keep your gaze soft and forward, focusing on a point in front of you.
- Engage your abdominal muscles to support your lower back.
- Ground down through all four corners of your feet to feel stable and rooted.

2. Cat-Cow Stretch

Guidelines:

- Start on your hands and knees in a tabletop position, wrists under shoulders and knees under hips.
- Inhale, arch your back, lift your chest and tailbone (Cow Pose).
- Exhale, round your spine, tuck your chin towards your chest (Cat Pose).
- Flow smoothly between Cat and Cow poses with each breath.

Benefits:

- Improves spinal flexibility and mobility.

- Releases tension in the back, neck, and shoulders.
- Stimulates the digestive organs and massages the internal organs.

Tips:

- Move slowly and mindfully, focusing on the movement of your spine.
- Coordinate your breath with the movement: inhale for Cow Pose, exhale for Cat Pose.
- Keep your movements fluid and gentle, avoiding any strain or discomfort.

3. Downward Facing Dog (Adho Mukha Svanasana)

Guidelines:

- Start in a tabletop position, then tuck your toes and lift your hips towards the ceiling.
- Press your hands firmly into the mat, arms straight and shoulder-width apart.

℘ Lengthen through your spine, straighten your legs, and press your heels towards the floor.

℘ Relax your head and neck, keeping your gaze towards your feet or belly button.

Benefits:

- Stretches the entire body, including the back, hamstrings, calves, and shoulders.
- Strengthens the arms, shoulders, and core muscles.
- Calms the mind and relieves stress and fatigue.

Tips:

- Keep a slight bend in your knees if your hamstrings are tight.
- Spread your fingers wide and press down through the knuckles to distribute weight evenly.
- Lift your sit bones towards the ceiling to lengthen through your spine.

4. Warrior I (Virabhadrasana I)

Guidelines:

- ℘ Start in a standing position at the top of your mat.
- ℘ Step your left foot back and turn it out at a 45-degree angle, keeping your right foot forward.
- ℘ Bend your right knee to stack it over your right ankle, with your thigh parallel to the floor.
- ℘ Reach your arms overhead, palms facing each other, and gaze towards your fingertips.

Benefits:

- Strengthens the legs, glutes, and core muscles.
- Opens the hips and chest, improving flexibility and range of motion.
- Builds confidence, courage, and inner strength.

Tips:

- Ground down through the outer edge of your back foot to stabilize your stance.
- Square your hips towards the front of the mat to deepen the stretch in the hip flexors.
- Lift through your torso and reach through your fingertips to lengthen your spine.

5. Warrior II (Virabhadrasana II)

Guidelines:

- From Warrior I, open your hips and arms parallel to the sides of the mat.
- Align your front heel with the arch of your back foot.
- Bend your front knee to stack it over your ankle, keeping your thigh parallel to the floor.
- Extend your arms out to the sides at shoulder height, palms facing down.

Benefits:

- Improves stamina, endurance, and concentration.

- Stretches the groin, hips, and chest muscles.
- Builds strength in the legs, arms, and shoulders.

Tips:

- Keep your shoulders relaxed and away from your ears.
- Engage your core muscles to support your lower back and maintain stability.
- Gaze over your front fingertips, keeping your neck long and aligned with your spine.

6. Tree Pose (Vrksasana)

Guidelines:

- Stand tall with your feet hip-width apart and arms by your sides.
- Shift your weight onto your left foot and lift your right foot off the ground.
- Place the sole of your right foot against your inner left thigh or calf, avoiding the knee.

∞ Bring your palms together at your heart
center or extend your arms overhead.

Benefits:

- Improves balance, coordination, and
  concentration.
- Strengthens the muscles of the legs, ankles,
  and feet.
- Stretches the hips, groin, and inner thighs.

Tips:

- Find a focal point to gaze at to help maintain
  balance and focus.
- Press your foot into your thigh or calf and
  your thigh back into your foot to create
  resistance.
- Keep your standing leg strong and engage
  your core to support your posture.

7. Cobra Pose (Bhujangasana)

Guidelines:

- Lie on your stomach with your palms flat on the mat under your shoulders.
- Press the tops of your feet into the mat and engage your leg muscles.
- Inhale, straighten your arms, and lift your chest off the mat, keeping your elbows close to your body.
- Lengthen through your spine and gaze forward, avoiding crunching your neck.

Benefits:

- Strengthens the muscles of the back, arms, and shoulders.
- Stretches the chest, abdomen, and front of the body.
- Improves posture and counteracts the effects of sitting and slouching.

Tips:

- Use your back muscles to lift your chest, rather than relying solely on your arms.
- Keep your shoulders relaxed and away from your ears, avoiding hunching.

-   Press down through the tops of your feet to protect your lower back.

8. Child's Pose (Balasana)

Guidelines:

- Kneel on the mat with your big toes touching and knees hip-width apart.
- Sit back on your heels and fold forward, resting your forehead on the mat.
- Extend your arms out in front of you or alongside your body, palms facing up.
- Relax your shoulders, soften your breath, and surrender to the pose.

Benefits:

-   Relaxes the body and calms the mind.
-   Stretches the hips, thighs, and ankles.
-   Relieves tension in the back, neck, and shoulders.

Tips:

- Use a bolster or folded blanket under your forehead for support if needed.
- Allow your belly to soften and sink towards the mat with each breath.
- Take slow, deep breaths and focus on releasing tension with each exhale.

9. Seated Forward Fold (Paschimottanasana)

Guidelines:

- Sit on the mat with your legs extended in front of you and feet flexed.
- Inhale, lengthen through your spine, and exhale, hinge at your hips to fold forward.
- Reach for your feet, shins, or thighs, keeping your back straight.
- Relax your neck, shoulders, and jaw, and breathe deeply into the stretch.

Benefits:

- Stretches the hamstrings, calves, and lower back.
- Calms the mind and soothes stress and anxiety.

- Stimulates the abdominal organs and improves digestion.

Tips:

- Keep a slight bend in your knees if your hamstrings are tight.
- Lengthen your spine with each inhale and deepen the stretch with each exhale.
- Focus on folding from your hips rather than rounding your spine.

10. Corpse Pose (Savasana)

Guidelines:

- Lie on your back with your legs extended and arms by your sides, palms facing up.
- Close your eyes and relax your entire body, letting go of tension and effort.
- Allow your breath to return to its natural rhythm and observe the sensations in your body.
- Remain in Savasana for 5-10 minutes, soaking in the benefits of your practice.

Benefits:

- Relaxes the body and calms the nervous system.
- Reduces stress, anxiety, and fatigue.
- Integrates the benefits of your yoga practice and promotes deep relaxation.

Tips:

- Use props such as blankets, bolsters, or eye pillows for added comfort and support.
- Scan your body from head to toe, consciously releasing any tension or tightness.
- Surrender completely to the present moment, letting go of thoughts and distractions.

11. Bridge Pose (Setu Bandhasana)

Guidelines:

- Lie on your back with your knees bent and feet hip-width apart, arms by your sides.
- Press your feet into the mat, engage your glutes, and lift your hips towards the ceiling.

- Interlace your hands under your back and roll your shoulders underneath you.
- Keep your neck long and gaze towards the ceiling.

Benefits:

- Strengthens the back, glutes, and hamstrings.
- Stretches the chest, neck, and spine.
- Improves posture and relieves lower back pain.

Tips:

- Press down through your feet evenly to lift your hips higher.
- Engage your core muscles to support your lower back.
- Relax your jaw and facial muscles to release tension.

12. Extended Triangle Pose (Utthita Trikonasana)

Guidelines:

- Stand at the top of your mat with your feet wide apart, toes pointing forward.
- Extend your arms out to the sides at shoulder height.
- Turn your right foot out 90 degrees and your left foot slightly inwards.
- Reach your right hand towards your right foot, placing it on your shin, ankle, or the floor.
- Extend your left arm towards the ceiling, stacking your shoulders.

Benefits:

- Stretches the hamstrings, hips, and groins.
- Strengthens the legs, core, and spine.
- Improves balance, stability, and concentration.

Tips:

- Keep your chest open and shoulders stacked to avoid collapsing forward.
- Engage your quadriceps to stabilize your front leg.
- Gaze towards your top hand or down towards the floor for balance.

13. Warrior III (Virabhadrasana III)

Guidelines:

- Begin in Mountain Pose (Tadasana) at the top of your mat.
- Shift your weight onto your right foot and hinge forward at your hips.
- Extend your left leg straight back behind you, parallel to the floor.
- Reach your arms forward alongside your ears, palms facing each other.

Benefits:

- Strengthens the legs, core, and shoulders.
- Improves balance, coordination, and proprioception.
- Builds confidence and focus.

Tips:

- Keep your hips level and facing towards the floor.
- Engage your core to stabilize your torso and protect your lower back.

- Reach actively through your fingertips and
  toes to lengthen your body.

14. Garland Pose (Malasana)

Guidelines:

- ℘ Begin in a squat position with your feet
  slightly wider than hip-width apart, toes
  turned out.
- ℘ Lower your hips towards the floor, keeping
  your heels on the ground.
- ℘ Bring your palms together at your heart
  center and use your elbows to press your
  knees gently open.

Benefits:

- Opens the hips, groin, and inner thighs.
- Strengthens the legs, ankles, and feet.
- Improves mobility and flexibility in the
  lower body.

Tips:

- If your heels lift off the ground, place a folded blanket or block under them for support.
- Keep your spine long and chest lifted to avoid rounding forward.
- Press your elbows into your knees to deepen the stretch in the hips.

15. Puppy Pose (Uttana Shishosana)

Guidelines:

- Begin in a tabletop position with your wrists under your shoulders and knees under your hips.
- Walk your hands forward and lower your chest towards the mat, keeping your hips stacked over your knees.
- Lower your forehead or chin to the mat and relax your neck and shoulders.

Benefits:

- Stretches the spine, shoulders, and chest.
- Relieves tension in the upper back, neck, and shoulders.
- Calms the mind and promotes relaxation.

Tips:

- Keep your hips lifted and engage your core to protect your lower back.
- Press firmly into your palms and fingertips to create length in the spine.
- Breathe deeply into the stretch, focusing on expanding the chest and ribcage.

16. Butterfly Pose (Baddha Konasana)

Guidelines:

- Sit on the mat with your legs extended in front of you.
- Bend your knees and bring the soles of your feet together, allowing your knees to fall out to the sides.
- Hold onto your ankles or feet with your hands and sit up tall.
- Gently press your knees towards the mat to deepen the stretch.

- Benefits:
- Opens the hips, groin, and inner thighs.

- Stimulates the abdominal organs and improves digestion.
- Relieves tension and discomfort in the lower back and hips.

Tips:

- Keep your spine long and avoid rounding forward.
- Press your elbows into your inner thighs to deepen the stretch.
- Relax your shoulders and breathe deeply into the pose.

17. Extended Puppy Pose (Utthita Balasana)

Guidelines:

- Start in a tabletop position with your wrists under your shoulders and knees under your hips.
- Walk your hands forward and lower your chest towards the mat, keeping your hips stacked over your knees.
- Extend your arms forward and relax your forehead or chin to the mat.

Benefits:

- Stretches the spine, shoulders, and chest.
- Releases tension in the upper back, neck, and shoulders.
- Calms the mind and promotes relaxation.

Tips:

- Keep your hips lifted and engage your core to protect your lower back.
- Press firmly into your palms and fingertips to create length in the spine.
- Breathe deeply into the stretch, focusing on expanding the chest and ribcage.

18. Cobra Twist Pose (Bhujangasana Twist)

Guidelines:

- Lie on your stomach with your palms flat on the mat under your shoulders.
- Press the tops of your feet into the mat and engage your leg muscles.
- Inhale, straighten your arms, and lift your chest off the mat.

₰ Exhale, twist to the right, bringing your left hand to your right shoulder and looking over your right shoulder. Switch sides.

Benefits:

- Strengthens the muscles of the back, arms, and shoulders.
- Stretches the chest, abdomen, and front of the body.
- Improves posture and counteracts the effects of sitting and slouching.

Tips:

- Use your back muscles to lift your chest, rather than relying solely on your arms.
- Keep your shoulders relaxed and away from your ears, avoiding hunching.
- Press down through the tops of your feet to protect your lower back.

19. Seated Spinal Twist (Ardha Matsyendrasana)

Guidelines:

- Sit on the mat with your legs extended in front of you.
- Bend your right knee and cross it over your left leg, placing your right foot flat on the floor.
- Hug your right knee with your left arm and place your right hand on the mat behind your back.
- Inhale, lengthen through your spine, and exhale, twist to the right, looking over your right shoulder. Switch sides.

Benefits:

- Stretches the spine, shoulders, and hips.
- Stimulates the digestive organs and improves digestion.
- Relieves tension and discomfort in the back and shoulders.

Tips:

- Keep both sit bones grounded on the mat.
- Lengthen through your spine with each inhale, and deepen the twist with each exhale.
- Use your breath to create space and openness in the spine.

20. Corpse Pose (Savasana)

Guidelines:

- Lie on your back with your legs extended and arms by your sides, palms facing up.
- Close your eyes and relax your entire body, letting go of tension and effort.
- Allow your breath to return to its natural rhythm and observe the sensations in your body.
- Remain in Savasana for 5-10 minutes, soaking in the benefits of your practice.

Benefits:

- Relaxes the body and calms the nervous system.
- Reduces stress, anxiety, and fatigue.
- Integrates the benefits of your yoga practice and promotes deep relaxation.

Tips:

- Use props such as blankets, bolsters, or eye pillows for added comfort and support.

- Scan your body from head to toe, consciously releasing any tension or tightness.
- Surrender completely to the present moment, letting go of thoughts and distractions.

Incorporate these beginner-friendly yoga poses into your practice, focusing on proper alignment, mindful breathing, and listening to your body's cues. With consistent practice and patience, you'll gradually build strength, flexibility, and inner peace on your yoga journey.

Chapter 13: Yoga for Intermediates

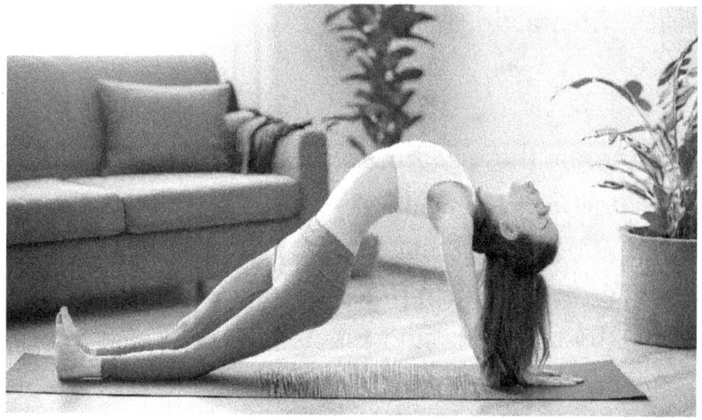

Incorporating these intermediate yoga poses into your practice can help you deepen your practice, build strength and flexibility, and cultivate mindfulness and presence on the mat. Remember to listen to your body, respect your limits, and approach each pose with curiosity and awareness. With consistent practice and patience, you'll continue to progress on your yoga journey and experience the transformative benefits of this ancient practice.

1. Warrior II (Virabhadrasana II)

Guidelines:

- Start in Mountain Pose (Tadasana).
- Step your feet wide apart, about 3-4 feet distance.
- Turn your right foot out 90 degrees and your left foot slightly inward. Bend your right knee to stack it directly over your ankle, keeping your left leg straight.
- Extend your arms parallel to the floor, with your shoulders relaxed away from your ears.
- Gaze over your right fingertips.

Benefits:

- Warrior II strengthens the legs, hips, and core muscles.
- It improves balance, stamina, and concentration.
- This pose also opens the hips and chest, enhancing flexibility and mobility.

Tips:

- Ensure your knee is aligned with your ankle and doesn't collapse inward.
- Keep your torso upright and engage your core to support the lower back.

- Press firmly through the outer edge of your
  back foot to maintain stability.

2. Triangle Pose (Trikonasana)

Guidelines:

- From Warrior II, straighten your right leg
  and reach your right arm forward, extending
  it over your right leg.
- Lower your right hand to your shin, ankle,
  or the floor, and extend your left arm up
  towards the ceiling.
- Keep your torso open and your gaze directed
  towards your left fingertips.

Benefits:

- Triangle Pose stretches the hamstrings, hips,
  and side body.
- It strengthens the legs, core, and spine while
  improving balance and stability.
- This pose also stimulates digestion and
  relieves lower back pain.

Tips:

- Engage your thigh muscles to support the lifted leg and avoid hyperextending the knee.
- Keep your chest and hips open towards the side, avoiding collapsing forward or backward.
- Use a block under your bottom hand if you cannot reach the floor comfortably.

3. Extended Side Angle Pose (Utthita Parsvakonasana)

Guidelines:

- From Warrior II, lower your right forearm to your right thigh and extend your left arm overhead, reaching towards the front of the room.
- Keep your right knee bent directly over your ankle and your torso extended forward.
- Lengthen through your side body and open your chest towards the ceiling.

Benefits:

- Extended Side Angle Pose strengthens the legs, hips, and core muscles.
- It stretches the side body, groin, and shoulders while improving flexibility and stability.
- This pose also stimulates digestion and increases circulation.

Tips:

- Press firmly through the outer edge of your back foot and engage your thigh muscles to stabilize the pose.
- Keep your spine long and avoid collapsing into the lower back.
- Use a block under your bottom hand if needed for support.

4. Revolved Triangle Pose (Parivrtta Trikonasana)

Guidelines:

- From Triangle Pose, place your left hand on the floor or a block outside your right foot.

- ℘ Extend your right arm up towards the ceiling, twisting your torso to the right.
- ℘ Keep your hips square and your gaze directed towards your right fingertips or towards the floor for balance.

Benefits:

- Revolved Triangle Pose strengthens the legs, core, and spine.
- It stretches the hamstrings, hips, and shoulders while improving balance and coordination.
- This pose also stimulates the abdominal organs and aids in detoxification.

Tips:

- Ground through the outer edge of your back foot and engage your thigh muscles to maintain stability.
- Keep your chest open and avoid collapsing into the twist.
- Use a block under your bottom hand if you cannot reach the floor comfortably.

5. Half Moon Pose (Ardha Chandrasana)

Guidelines:

- From Triangle Pose, bend your right knee and shift your weight onto your right foot.
- Place your left hand on your left hip and extend your right fingertips forward, about a foot in front of your right foot.
- Lift your left leg parallel to the floor, flexing your left foot.
- Open your hips and chest towards the left side, and extend your left arm up towards the ceiling.

Benefits:

- Half Moon Pose strengthens the legs, core, and ankles.
- It improves balance, concentration, and coordination while stretching the hamstrings, groins, and side body.
- This pose also stimulates the abdominal organs and improves digestion.

Tips:

- Use a block under your right hand for support if you cannot reach the floor comfortably.
- Engage your core muscles to support the lifted leg and maintain stability.
- Keep your hips and shoulders stacked vertically to the floor.

6. Camel Pose (Ustrasana)

Guidelines:

- Kneel on the mat with your knees hip-width apart and your thighs perpendicular to the floor.
- Place your hands on your lower back, fingers pointing downward. Inhale, lift your chest towards the ceiling, and gently arch your spine backward.
- Reach your hands towards your heels, keeping your hips stacked over your knees.

Benefits:

- Camel Pose stretches the front body, including the chest, abdomen, and hip flexors.

- It strengthens the back muscles and improves spinal flexibility and posture.
- This pose also stimulates the thyroid gland and boosts energy levels.

Tips:

- Press your shins and the tops of your feet firmly into the mat to stabilize the pose.
- Engage your core muscles to support your lower back and avoid compressing the lumbar spine.
- Keep your neck long and gaze towards the ceiling or slightly behind you.

7. Crow Pose (Bakasana)

Guidelines:

- Start in a squat position with your feet hip-width apart and your palms shoulder-width apart on the mat.
- Bend your elbows slightly and lean forward, bringing your knees towards your upper arms.

℘ Shift your weight onto your hands, engage your core, and lift your feet off the mat, balancing on your hands.

Benefits:

- Crow Pose strengthens the arms, wrists, and core muscles.
- It improves balance, concentration, and coordination while building confidence and courage.
- This pose also stimulates the abdominal organs and boosts metabolism.

Tips:

- Keep your elbows slightly bent and hug them towards each other to create a stable foundation for the pose.
- Engage your core muscles and lift your hips high to shift the weight forward onto your hands.
- Gaze slightly forward to maintain balance and stability.

8. Wheel Pose (Urdhva Dhanurasana)

Guidelines:

- Lie on your back with your knees bent and feet hip-width apart, close to your hips.
- Place your hands beside your ears, fingers pointing towards your shoulders.
- Press into your hands and feet, lifting your hips towards the ceiling.
- Straighten your arms and legs, coming into a full backbend.

Benefits:

- Wheel Pose strengthens the arms, shoulders, back, and legs.
- It improves spinal flexibility, opens the chest and shoulders, and stimulates the nervous system.
- This pose also energizes the body and promotes a sense of vitality and well-being.

Tips:

- Engage your glutes and thighs to lift your hips higher and support your lower back.
- Keep your elbows parallel and avoid letting them splay out to the sides.

- Press firmly into your hands and feet to lift your chest towards the ceiling.

9. Flying Pigeon Pose (Eka Pada Galavasana)

Guidelines:

- Start in Downward Facing Dog.
- Lift your right leg high, then bend your right knee and draw it towards your chest.
- Place your right knee on your right tricep or upper arm.
- Lean forward, shift your weight onto your hands, and engage your core. Extend your left leg back and up, straightening it behind you.

Benefits:

- Flying Pigeon Pose strengthens the arms, shoulders, core, and hip flexors.
- It improves balance, concentration, and hip mobility while building strength and stability.

-   This pose also requires mental focus and perseverance.

Tips:

-   Begin with low Flying Pigeon variations, such as keeping the back foot on the mat or using a block under the hands for support.
-   Engage your core and hug your elbows towards each other to create stability in the pose.
-   Keep your gaze focused and breathe deeply to maintain balance.

10. Forearm Stand (Pincha Mayurasana)

Guidelines:

-   Start in Dolphin Pose, with your forearms on the mat, elbows shoulder-width apart, and fingers interlaced.
-   Walk your feet closer to your elbows, coming into a dolphin plank position.
-   Lift one leg towards the ceiling, then kick up with the other leg, coming into a forearm stand.

℘ Keep your core engaged and your gaze focused between your forearms.

Benefits:

- Forearm Stand strengthens the arms, shoulders, core, and back muscles.
- It improves balance, concentration, and upper body strength while increasing blood flow to the brain.
- This pose also boosts confidence and mental clarity.

Tips:

- Practice forearm strength-building exercises, such as Dolphin Pose and Dolphin Plank, to prepare for Forearm Stand.
- Use a wall for support and practice kicking up lightly to find balance.
- Engage your core and legs to lift the hips higher and maintain stability in the pose.

11. Firefly Pose (Tittibhasana)

Guidelines:

- Start in a squatting position with your feet slightly wider than hip-width apart.
- Place your hands on the floor between your feet, fingers pointing forward.
- Shift your weight onto your hands, bend your elbows slightly, and lift your feet off the ground.
- Extend your legs out to the sides, straightening them as much as possible.

Benefits:

- Firefly Pose strengthens the arms, wrists, core, and inner thighs.
- It improves balance, concentration, and hip flexibility while toning the abdominal muscles and improving digestion.
- This pose also requires mental focus and stability.

Tips:

- Begin by practicing variations of the pose, such as lifting one foot at a time or using blocks under the hands for support.

- Engage your core muscles and press firmly through your palms to lift the hips and legs off the ground.
- Keep your chest lifted and gaze forward to maintain balance.

12. Side Crow Pose (Parsva Bakasana)

Guidelines:

- Start in a squatting position with your feet hip-width apart.
- Place your hands on the mat shoulder-width apart, fingers spread wide.
- Shift your weight onto your hands, bend your elbows, and lean forward, bringing your knees to the outside of your upper arms.
- Engage your core and lift your feet off the ground, balancing on your hands.

Benefits:

- Side Crow Pose strengthens the arms, wrists, core, and oblique.
- It improves balance, concentration, and upper body strength while toning the

abdominal muscles and improving
coordination.
- This pose also stimulates digestion and
detoxification.

Tips:

- Begin by practicing Crow Pose to build
strength and confidence before attempting
Side Crow.
- Keep your elbows bent and hug them
towards each other to create a stable
foundation for the pose.
- Engage your core muscles and gaze forward
to maintain balance and stability.

13. Eight-Angle Pose (Astavakrasana)

Guidelines:

- Start in a seated position with your legs
extended in front of you.
- Bend your right knee and place your right
foot on the floor outside your left thigh.
- Thread your right arm under your right leg
and clasp your hands together.

- ℘ Lean forward, shift your weight onto your hands, and lift your hips off the ground.
- ℘ Extend your left leg out to the side and straighten both arms, balancing on your hands.

Benefits:

- Eight-Angle Pose strengthens the arms, wrists, core, and hip flexors.
- It improves balance, concentration, and upper body strength while toning the abdominal muscles and improving flexibility.
- This pose also stimulates digestion and detoxification.

Tips:

- Begin by practicing preparatory poses, such as seated twists and arm balances, to prepare the body for Eight-Angle Pose.
- Engage your core muscles and press firmly through your palms to lift the hips and legs off the ground.
- Keep your chest lifted and gaze forward to maintain balance.

14. Flying Lizard Pose (Dvi Pada Galavasana)

Guidelines:

- Start in Downward Facing Dog.
- Lift your right leg high, then bend your right knee and draw it towards your right tricep or upper arm. Lean forward, shift your weight onto your hands, and engage your core.
- Extend your left leg back and up, straightening it behind you.
- Hook your left foot around your right ankle or calf, coming into a twisted arm balance.

Benefits:

- Flying Lizard Pose strengthens the arms, shoulders, core, and hip flexors.
- It improves balance, concentration, and hip mobility while building strength and stability.
- This pose also requires mental focus and perseverance.

Tips:

- Begin with low Flying Lizard variations, such as keeping the back foot on the mat or using a block under the hands for support.
- Engage your core and hug your elbows towards each other to create stability in the pose.
- Keep your gaze focused and breathe deeply to maintain balance.

15. Grasshopper Pose (Parivrtta Bhekasana)

Guidelines:

- Start lying on your stomach with your chin on the mat.
- Bend your knees and reach back with your hands to grab the outsides of your feet.
- Lift your chest and head off the mat as you kick your feet into your hands.
- Press into your hands and lift your feet towards the ceiling, coming into a backbend with your legs extended overhead.

Benefits:

- Grasshopper Pose strengthens the back muscles, shoulders, and legs.

- It improves spinal flexibility, opens the chest and shoulders, and stimulates the abdominal organs.
- This pose also improves posture and boosts energy levels.

Tips:

- Engage your core muscles and press your thighs together to stabilize the pose.
- Keep your neck long and gaze forward to avoid compressing the cervical spine.
- Use a strap or towel to reach your feet if you cannot grab them with your hands.

16. One-Legged King Pigeon Pose (Eka Pada Rajakapotasana)

Guidelines:

- Start in Downward Facing Dog.
- Lift your right leg high, then bend your right knee and draw it towards your chest.
- Place your right knee behind your right wrist and your right foot behind your left wrist.
- Slide your left leg back, keeping your hips square.

⨏ Lower down onto your forearms or extend your arms forward, folding over your front leg.

Benefits:

- One-Legged King Pigeon Pose stretches the hip flexors, quadriceps, and hip rotators.
- It improves hip mobility, opens the chest and shoulders, and stimulates the abdominal organs.
- This pose also releases tension in the lower back and promotes relaxation.

Tips:

- Use props such as blocks or blankets under your hips or forearms for support if needed.
- Keep your hips level and square to the front of the mat to maintain alignment.
- Relax your neck and shoulders, and breathe deeply into the pose.

17. Bound Side Angle Pose (Baddha Parsvakonasana)

Guidelines:

- From Warrior II, lower your right hand to the inside of your right foot.
- Reach your left arm behind your back and clasp your hands together, binding your arms.
- Sink your hips lower, bringing your torso towards the inside of your right thigh.
- Keep your chest and hips open, and gaze towards the ceiling.

Benefits:

- Bound Side Angle Pose strengthens the legs, hips, and core muscles.
- It improves balance, concentration, and shoulder flexibility while stretching the side body and groins.
- This pose also stimulates digestion and detoxification.

Tips:

- Use a strap or towel to bridge the gap between your hands if you cannot clasp them together.
- Press firmly through the outer edge of your back foot and engage your thigh muscles to stabilize the pose.

- Keep your chest lifted and gaze upward to deepen the stretch.

18. Revolved Half Moon Pose (Parivrtta Ardha Chandrasana)

Guidelines:

- From Half Moon Pose, bend your left knee and reach your left hand towards the floor or a block.
- Extend your right arm up towards the ceiling and rotate your torso to the left, stacking your shoulders and opening your chest towards the ceiling.
- Keep your hips level and your gaze directed towards your right fingertips.

Benefits:

- Revolved Half Moon Pose strengthens the legs, core, and shoulders.
- It improves balance, concentration, and spinal mobility while stretching the hamstrings, hips, and side body.

- This pose also stimulates digestion and detoxification.

Tips:

- Use a block under your bottom hand for support if you cannot reach the floor comfortably.
- Engage your core muscles and press firmly through your standing foot to maintain stability.
- Keep your chest open and gaze upward to deepen the twist.

19. Standing Split Pose (Urdhva Prasarita Eka Padasana)

Guidelines:

- From Warrior III, bend your left knee slightly and shift your weight onto your right foot.
- Bring your hands to the mat on either side of your right foot and begin to straighten your right leg.

℘ Lift your left leg towards the ceiling, extending it as high as possible while keeping your hips square.

℘ Flex your right foot and engage your core to support the pose.

Benefits:

- Standing Split Pose strengthens the legs, core, and hip flexors.
- It improves balance, concentration, and hamstring flexibility while stretching the calves and Achilles tendon.
- This pose also energizes the body and promotes a sense of lightness and buoyancy.

Tips:

- Keep your standing leg strong and engage your glutes to stabilize the pose.
- Use blocks under your hands for support if you cannot reach the floor comfortably.
- Keep your hips level and avoid collapsing into the standing hip.
- Flex your lifted foot and point your toes towards the ceiling to deepen the stretch.

20. Scorpion Pose (Vrischikasana)

Guidelines:

- Start in Downward Facing Dog. Lift your right leg high, then bend your knee and draw it towards your chest.
- Begin to arch your back and kick your right foot towards your head, allowing your heel to come towards your upper back.
- Press into your hands and lift your chest towards the ceiling, coming into a backbend with your head lifted off the mat.

Benefits:

- Scorpion Pose strengthens the arms, shoulders, back, and core muscles.
- It improves spinal flexibility, opens the chest and shoulders, and stimulates the nervous system.
- This pose also requires mental focus and concentration.

Tips:

- Practice preparatory poses such as Downward Facing Dog, Upward Facing Dog, and Camel Pose to warm up and prepare the body for Scorpion Pose.
- Engage your core muscles and press firmly through your palms to lift your chest towards the ceiling.
- Keep your neck long and gaze forward to maintain balance and stability.

Chapter 14: Health Enhancement Techniques

In this chapter, we delve into various health enhancement techniques that complement and support your yoga practice. These techniques are designed to optimize your physical, mental, and emotional well-being, providing you with additional tools to enhance your overall health and vitality.

1. Meditation

Guidance:

- Meditation involves training the mind to focus and redirect thoughts, leading to increased awareness, clarity, and inner peace.
- Find a quiet and comfortable space, close your eyes, and focus on your breath or a specific mantra or visualization.

Benefits:

- Regular meditation practice reduces stress, anxiety, and depression while improving concentration, emotional balance, and overall mental health.
- It promotes relaxation, enhances self-awareness, and cultivates a sense of inner tranquility and equanimity.

Tips:

- Start with short meditation sessions of 5-10 minutes and gradually increase the duration as you become more comfortable.
- Experiment with different meditation techniques to find what works best for you, whether it's mindfulness meditation, loving-kindness meditation, or guided visualization.

2. Pranayama (Breath Control)

Guidance:

- Pranayama techniques involve conscious control and regulation of the breath to promote physical, mental, and emotional well-being.
- Practice deep breathing, alternate nostril breathing (Nadi Shodhana), or Kapalabhati (skull shining breath) to purify and energize the body.

Benefits:

- Pranayama practice increases lung capacity, improves respiratory function, and enhances oxygenation of the blood and tissues.

- It calms the nervous system, reduces stress and anxiety, and promotes mental clarity and focus.

Tips:

- Start with simple pranayama techniques and gradually progress to more advanced practices as you gain experience.
- Practice pranayama in a comfortable seated position with a straight spine, and focus on smooth, steady breaths.
- Consult with a qualified yoga instructor for personalized guidance and instruction.

3. Yoga Nidra (Yogic Sleep)

Guidance:

- Yoga Nidra is a guided relaxation technique that induces a state of deep relaxation and conscious sleep.
- Lie down in Savasana (corpse pose), close your eyes, and follow the instructions of the guided meditation as you systematically relax each part of your body.

Benefits:

-   Yoga Nidra promotes deep relaxation, stress
    relief, and rejuvenation at the physical,
    mental, and emotional levels.
-   It enhances sleep quality, reduces insomnia,
    and alleviates symptoms of anxiety,
    depression, and PTSD.

Tips:

-   Practice Yoga Nidra regularly, especially
    before bedtime or during times of
    heightened stress or fatigue.
-   Find a quiet and comfortable space where
    you won't be disturbed, and use headphones
    to enhance the audio experience of guided
    meditations.
-   Explore different Yoga Nidra recordings to
    find ones that resonate with you.

4. Ayurveda (Yoga's Sister Science)

Guidance:

- Ayurveda is a holistic healing system that originated in India thousands of years ago.
- It emphasizes the importance of balancing the mind, body, and spirit through diet, lifestyle, and herbal remedies based on individual constitution (dosha).

Benefits:

- Ayurveda offers personalized guidance for optimizing health and well-being, including recommendations for dietary choices, daily routines, and self-care practices.
- It addresses imbalances and ailments at their root cause, promoting holistic healing and longevity.

Tips:

- Learn about your unique Ayurvedic constitution (dosha) and follow dietary and lifestyle recommendations tailored to your specific needs.
- Incorporate Ayurvedic practices such as daily self-massage (abhyanga), oil pulling, and herbal supplementation to support overall health and vitality.

- Consult with an Ayurvedic practitioner for personalized assessment and guidance.

5. Mindful Eating

Guidance:

- Mindful eating involves cultivating awareness and attention while eating, focusing on the sensory experience of food and tuning into hunger and fullness cues.
- Slow down, savor each bite, and pay attention to the taste, texture, and aroma of your food.

Benefits:

- Mindful eating promotes healthier eating habits, prevents overeating, and improves digestion and nutrient absorption.

-   It fosters a deeper connection with food and fosters gratitude, enjoyment, and satisfaction with meals.

Tips:

-   Practice mindful eating by turning off distractions such as screens and phones during meals, chewing slowly and thoroughly, and engaging all your senses in the eating experience.
-   Tune into hunger and fullness signals, and honor your body's natural cues for nourishment and satisfaction.

6. Self-Myofascial Release (SMR)

Guidance:

-   Self-myofascial release involves using tools such as foam rollers, massage balls, or massage sticks to apply pressure to tight or restricted areas of muscle and connective tissue (fascia).

- ℘ Roll or massage the targeted areas with gentle pressure, focusing on areas of tension or discomfort.

Benefits:

- SMR helps release tension, knots, and adhesions in the muscles and fascia, promoting increased flexibility, range of motion, and muscle recovery.
- It improves circulation, reduces muscle soreness, and enhances overall mobility and performance.

Tips:

- Incorporate SMR into your pre and post-yoga routines to prepare the body for movement and aid in recovery.
- Start with gentle pressure and gradually increase intensity as tolerated.
- Focus on major muscle groups such as the calves, quadriceps, hamstrings, glutes, and upper back.

7. Hydration

Guidance:

- ℘ Hydration is essential for overall health and well-being, including optimal bodily function, nutrient absorption, and toxin elimination.
- ℘ Drink an adequate amount of water throughout the day, aiming for at least 8-10 glasses of water or more depending on individual needs and activity levels.

Benefits:

- Proper hydration supports joint lubrication, muscle function, and cognitive performance.
- It maintains electrolyte balance, regulates body temperature, and promotes healthy digestion and detoxification.
- Hydration also enhances skin health and appearance.

Tips:

- Stay hydrated by drinking water regularly throughout the day, especially before, during, and after yoga practice.
- Monitor urine color to gauge hydration status, aiming for pale yellow to clear urine.

- Consider electrolyte-rich beverages such as coconut water or electrolyte supplements for enhanced hydration, particularly during intense physical activity.

8. Restorative Yoga

Guidance:

- Restorative yoga involves passive, supported poses held for extended periods to promote deep relaxation, stress relief, and rejuvenation.
- Use props such as bolsters, blankets, and blocks to support the body in comfortable, fully relaxed positions.

Benefits:

- Restorative yoga calms the nervous system, reduces stress hormones, and promotes physical and mental relaxation.
- It enhances flexibility, circulation, and immune function while reducing muscle tension, fatigue, and anxiety.

Tips:

- Practice restorative yoga as part of your evening wind-down routine or whenever you need to de-stress and unwind.
- Set up a quiet, dimly lit space with soft music or guided meditation to enhance the relaxation experience.
- Focus on slow, deep breathing and allow yourself to fully surrender into each pose.

9. Nature Immersion (Shinrin-Yoku)

Guidance:

- Nature immersion, also known as forest bathing or Shinrin-Yoku, involves spending time in natural environments to promote relaxation, stress reduction, and overall well-being.
- Take leisurely walks in parks, forests, or natural settings, engaging your senses and connecting with the natural world.

Benefits:

- Nature immersion reduces cortisol levels, lowers blood pressure, and boosts mood and immunity.
- It enhances mental clarity, creativity, and emotional resilience while fostering a sense of awe, wonder, and interconnectedness with nature.

Tips:

- Make time to immerse yourself in nature regularly, even if it's just for a short walk or outdoor meditation session.
- Leave behind distractions such as phones or electronic devices and fully engage your senses in the sights, sounds, smells, and textures of the natural environment.
- Practice mindfulness and gratitude for the healing power of nature.

10. Journaling and Reflection

Guidance:

- Journaling and reflection involve writing down thoughts, feelings, experiences, and

insights to gain clarity, self-awareness, and
personal growth.

- Set aside dedicated time each day to journal,
either in the morning to set intentions or in
the evening to reflect on the day's events.

Benefits:

- Journaling promotes self-expression,
emotional processing, and stress relief.
- It enhances self-awareness, problem-solving
skills, and goal-setting abilities while
fostering mindfulness, gratitude, and
positive thinking.
- Journaling also serves as a valuable tool for
tracking progress, insights, and personal
growth.

Tips:

- Keep a journal handy and write freely
without judgment or censorship.
- Experiment with different journaling
prompts, such as gratitude lists, daily
reflections, or goal-setting exercises.
- Use journaling as a means of self-discovery,
self-care, and self-expression, allowing it to

become a sacred space for reflection and growth.

By integrating these additional health enhancement techniques into your yoga practice and daily routine, you can further support your overall well-being and cultivate a balanced and harmonious lifestyle. Embrace these practices with openness and curiosity, and tailor them to suit your individual needs and preferences. Remember that wellness is a holistic journey, and each of these techniques offers valuable tools for nurturing your body, mind, and spirit.

Chapter 15:

Conclusion

As we reach the conclusion of "Yoga at Home: A Comprehensive Guide to 60 Plus Poses for Beginners and Intermediates, Including Benefits, Tips, and Health Enhancement Techniques" it's essential to reflect on the journey we've embarked on together and the profound impact that yoga can have on our lives.

Throughout this book, we've explored yoga, from its ancient roots in India to its global popularity as a holistic practice for physical, mental, and spiritual well-being. We've delved into the various types of yoga, beginner and intermediate poses, health enhancement techniques, and tips for establishing a home yoga practice.

Our exploration has revealed that yoga is not just a series of physical postures but a transformative journey of self-discovery, self-care, and self-realization. It is a practice that invites us to cultivate awareness, presence, and mindfulness in every aspect of our lives, both on and off the mat.

By embracing yoga as a way of life, we can experience a myriad of benefits, including improved strength, flexibility, balance, and vitality, as well as enhanced mental clarity, emotional resilience, and inner peace. Yoga offers us a path to holistic health and wellness, empowering us to live authentically, joyfully, and harmoniously.

As you continue your yoga journey beyond the pages of this book, I encourage you to approach your practice with an open heart and an open mind. Remember that yoga is a personal and ever-evolving practice, and there is no one-size-fits-all approach. Listen to your body, honor your limitations, and celebrate your progress, however small it may seem.

Whether you're a beginner taking your first steps on the yoga path or an experienced practitioner deepening your practice, may you find inspiration, guidance, and empowerment in the teachings shared within these pages. May your yoga journey be filled with grace, gratitude, and growth, leading you towards greater health, happiness, and wholeness.

Thank you for joining me on this transformative odyssey through the world of yoga. May your practice continue to illuminate your path and nourish your body, mind, and spirit for years to come.

Namaste.

www.ingramcontent.com/pod-product-compliance
Lightning Source LLC
Chambersburg PA
CBHW070757260726
48660CB00005B/1656